How to Cure Candida

Yeast Infection Causes, Symptoms,

Diet & Natural Remedies

By

Kelly Wallace

I0427137

Books by Kelly Wallace

———

10 MINUTES A DAY TO A Powerful New Life

Become Your Higher Self – Using Spiritual Energy to Transform Your Life

Chakras – Heal, Clear, And Strengthen Your Energy Centers

Clear Your Karma – The Healing Power of Your Past Lives

Contacting and Working with Your Angels

Contacting Your Spirit Guides – Meeting and Working with Your Invisible Helpers

Creating A Charmed Life – Enchantments to Attract, Repel, Cleanse & Heal

Energy Work – Heal, Cleanse, and Strengthen Your Aura

Everyday Miracles – Powerful Steps to Wonderful Experiences

Healing the Child Within – Rewrite Your Early Childhood Life Script

How to Cure Candida – Yeast Infection Symptoms, Causes, Diet & Natural Remedies

Intuitive Living – Developing Your Psychic Gifts

Intuitive Tarot – Learn the Tarot Instantly

Master the Art of Picking Up Women

Master the Art of Dating Women

Master the Art of Sex and Seduction

No-Sweat Homeschooling – The Cheap, Free, and Low-Stress Way to Teach Your Kids

Psychic Vampires – Protect and Heal Yourself from Energy Predators

Reprogram Your Subconscious – Use the Power of Your Mind

Spiritual Alchemy – Transform Your Life and Everyone In It

The Art of Happiness – Living A Life of Peace and Simplicity

The Love You Deserve – Releasing Toxic Relationships and Attracting Your Soulmate

The Power of Pets – How to Psychically Communicate with Your Pet

Transforming Your Money Mindset – From Broke To Abundance

True Wealth – Reprogram Your Subconscious for Financial Success

Upgrade Your Life – Small Changes, Easy Actions, Big Success

About Kelly Wallace

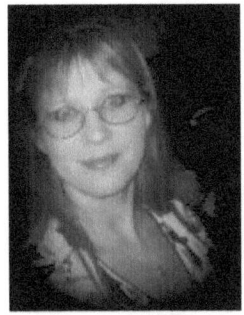

KELLY IS A BESTSELLING spiritual and self-help author, former radio show host, and has been a professional psychic counselor for over twenty years. She can see, hear, sense, and feel information sent from Spirit, the Universe, and a client's Higher Self.

Whether your problems or concerns center on love, finances, family, career, health, education, or your purpose in life, she writes books that will help you easily make lasting changes.

Kelly also offers professional psychic counseling, caring guidance, and solutions that work! More than just a typical psychic reading or counseling session, you will feel you've found a real friend during your time of need—whether you simply want answers and guidance to your current worries or concerns, or you're interested in learning more about your soulmate, spirit guides, angels, past lives, or anything else.

Contact her today for an in-depth and life-altering reading!

Website: DrKellyPsychic.com

Email: Dr.Kelly.Psychic.Counselor@gmail.com

What We'll Cover

———

A Silent Epidemic

———

I STRUGGLED WITH CANDIDA for years before finally curing myself. After going through my own frustrating experience, and talking to friends and clients who shared the same problem, I started doing more research on the subject.

I was surprised to discover that this fungus may affect up to 70% of the population, and accounts for nearly 7% of all hospital stays. Yet, most people aren't aware they have it. The symptoms are so wide and varied, leaving its victims feeling chronically ill with seemingly no cure.

Most mainstream doctors are uneducated about Candida and its impact on their patients' health. People can't find answers and go from doctor to doctor trying to find relief from their symptoms.

This is exactly what I went through for years. I felt exhausted, couldn't think clearly, had mood swings you wouldn't believe, food allergies, and even sex became painful—not that I had a libido at that point anyway!

I went to one doctor after another trying to find out what was wrong with me, spent too much money on tests, only to have each doctor shrug and take a wild guess as to what the problem was. I heard everything from, "It's all in your mind," to, "Chronic PMS." At one point I was told it was anemia and given regular B12 injections.

Obviously, none of this helped. I knew I wasn't crazy, though I sure felt like it at times. So, I went in search of my own cure.

After extensive online reading and poring over stacks of books, I finally realized I had systemic Candida and would, in time, be well again. It was a long journey, though it didn't need to be, which is why I wrote this book.

I want to save you time, money, and frustration by sharing in these pages common causes, symptoms, remedies, resources and more so you can decide (hopefully with the support and help of your physician) if Candida is robbing you of your health, and how to get well again.

There are many books written about Candida, though most of the authors haven't been where I was or where you are now. They simply gather information, put it in a book, and that's that. I know what you're going through and will discuss what worked for me, what didn't, and what I encountered.

This way, you'll be able to make educated choices for yourself and know somebody else has really been there and done that. A friend offering support that's come from real life experience.

Now, let's get you well!

What Is Candida Albicans?

———

THIS YEAST IS NATURALLY present in every human body, and is a normal part of your gut flora—a group of microorganisms that live in your digestive tract. When all conditions are just right, it causes no problem, but once things are out of balance though this yeast organism multiplies at lightning speed and takes over the healthy microorganisms.

You'd be surprised at how easy it is to throw this balance off and have Candida begin wreaking havoc. No wonder so many people are affected yet don't know it.

Where is this yeast usually found?

As I just mentioned, it's normally found in the digestive tract, but other places where this yeast normally grows are in the mouth, throat, and genitals. When out of control it can burrow into the intestines and enter the blood stream, making its way into your organs.

In my case, this is what I believe happened. Since the Candida went undetected for so long it had many, many months to multiply and take over.

Candida albicans emits seventy different toxins that leach into the body, which is why its victims feel so awful. You may think you have the flu, PMS, Chronic Fatigue Syndrome, or something worse.

No matter what you do, the symptoms won't go away. That's because we've been treating the symptoms rather than the root cause of the problem. But, if you don't know what the problem is in the first place, you're left to grope around in the dark hoping something somewhere will work. It can be so frustrating!

What happens once it takes over?

As the yeast multiplies and takes over the body, it causes a long list of chronic conditions and illnesses. Here are of some of the most common symptoms:

- abdominal gas

- headaches

- migraines

- excessive fatigue

- cravings for alcohol

- anxiety

- vaginitis

- rectal itching

- cravings for sweets

- fuzzy thinking

- inability to concentrate

- hyperactivity

- mood swings

- diarrhea

- constipation

- itchy skin

- acne

- eczema

- depression

- sinus inflammation

- PMS

- dizziness

- poor memory

- persistent cough

- earaches

- low sex drive

- muscle weakness

- irritability

- learning difficulties

- sensitivity to fragrances and/or other chemicals

- thrush

- athletes foot

- sore throat

- indigestion

- acid reflux

These are the main symptoms Candida sufferers experience, though the list is much longer than this. And, other illnesses or conditions can have many of these symptoms as well.

I had just a about everything on that list, but once I got the Candida under control, they all but disappeared! I couldn't remember how long it had been since I felt "normal."

After you look over the above list, if you find that you have three or more of the symptoms, make an appointment with your doctor to discuss the possibility of a Candida overgrowth and get tested. Later, I'll show you a simple home test you can do to see if you may have a yeast overgrowth.

Although Candida is difficult to eliminate from the body, highly effective treatments *are* available. Even home treatment works well, which is what I opted for. I try to stay away from prescription drugs as much as possible. Also, there are many people without insurance or have huge deductibles and co-pays. Treating Candida at home can be a sensible decision.

The protocol is actually very healthy and can eliminate other chronic health problems as well. I was amazed at the increase in my energy, mood, mental focus, and I even lost stubborn weight.

Candida Causes

———

ALTHOUGH THIS FUNGUS naturally lives in the gut, not causing any problems at all, things can easily trigger an overgrowth. Once this yeast is out of control, it quickly affects your entire system. Let's look at some of the most common causes of Candida takeover:

Stress

Stress can damage every part of a person; from their emotional state to their mind and body. It's also a common trigger for a Candida overgrowth, and who isn't under a lot of stress at times?

Factors such as a job, kids, school, finances, poor sleeping and eating habits, and relationship issues are all common stressors in life. When a person is stressed, it throws the body out of balance and opens the door for this fungus to grow like wildfire. A weakened body is an excellent breeding ground for yeast.

Humidity

As a fungus, Candida spreads quickly when heat and humidity are present. If you live in a humid climate such as is found in the Southern parts of the United States in summer, you could be more susceptible to Candida than those who live in drier climates.

When I lived in Baltimore I suffered with Candida constantly. However, once I moved to Tucson I had far fewer symptoms and could easily get it under control if it did pop up. Now that I'm living in Maryland again I pay close attention to even the smallest indicator that this infection might be coming back.

Of course, not everyone can or would want to move to a desert state like Arizona, New Mexico, or parts of California or Texas. Just be aware that if you live in a place with high humidity you'll need to work harder at healing any Candida overgrowth and keeping it at bay.

The Pill

Birth control pills are another trigger. The gut contains certain amounts of microorganisms and yeast that help to digest food, but the estrogen in birth control pills can throw off the body's natural hormonal balance. Once this happens, it's easy for the Candida fungus to take over.

Antibiotics

This is a huge culprit. Many people take long treatments of antibiotics for everything from acne to a strep infection. Doctors hand out antibiotic prescriptions like candy.

The problem is that antibiotics not only kill off the harmful bacteria causing the illness or acne breakout, but it also wipes out the beneficial bacteria living in the digestive tract. Once the good bacteria in the body are eliminated, the immune system is defenseless against the quickly growing yeast.

If you or a loved go through a course of antibiotics, it's good to follow a Candida health plan for a month or so, just to be sure your system gets back on track and to avoid a yeast breakout.

Sugars

Candida is yeast and yeast feeds off sugars. Drinking alcohol, eating a lot of starchy foods, and consuming foods with sugar all feed the yeast, allowing it to grow quickly. This even goes for natural sugars like honey, agave, or molasses.

Stress, humidity, birth control pills, antibiotics, and sugar all have a hand in causing a Candida overgrowth. It's no wonder so many people are probably affected by this fungus! Once the Candida grows and spreads, it releases toxins into the body and bloodstream leading to the symptoms listed above.

Men Can Get Yeast Infections

———

WHEN YOU HEAR ABOUT yeast infections you probably only think women can get them. The fact is that both men and women can get Candida. Once this fungus is in your body it can be difficult to get rid of unless you're diligent and do it right. Left untreated, it can enter your intestinal tract and cause a whole host of other problems. It's better to take care of it right away.

Symptoms

Most commonly, men will notice a yeast infection of the penis first. If it isn't taken care of it can spread throughout the body, just as it does in women. If you're a man and have Candida, you may notice that your penis feels itchy, and the skin could be dry and bumpy. The head of your penis may feel very sensitive or even sore and inflamed. It's easy to mistake this usually harmless condition with an STD, though they aren't in the same category.

How Men Get Candida

The most common way for a man to get a yeast infection is by having intercourse with a woman who has Candida of the vagina. It's also possible to get a yeast infection from using the same bath towel your partner did if she has the infection.

Natural Cures

Although I go into detail on how to cure Candida later in the book, I want to offer some remedies men can follow. A few natural ways of combating a yeast infection would be to take grape-fruit seed tablets (not to be confused with grape seed) and add things like yogurt, apple cider vinegar and garlic to your daily diet.

For an external treatment you could add a few drops of tea tree oil to a tablespoon of olive oil and rub that on 2-3 times a day. The tea tree oil may sting at first since your penis skin is irritated, but it will soon takeaway the itching and eventually help it to heal.

Also, if your partner has a yeast infection, be sure she seeks out treatment too and use condoms when having intercourse until she's healed.

Testing Yourself

———

THERE ARE A VARIETY of tests practitioners use to diagnose yeast overgrowth such as stool tests, blood tests, and urine tests, though they aren't always reliable. They may or may not detect a Candida infection. I had numerous tests performed and Candida was never found, though it's obvious to me now that I had a huge case of it.

The simplest and most effective way to know if you have a yeast problem is by your symptoms. One of the most accurate tests is the written questionnaire you can find in Dr. Crook's book called *The Yeast Syndrome*. There are also reputable websites that offer free Candida questionnaires. I'll provide some suggestions in the resources area at the end of the book.

After going over the list of symptoms we talked about earlier, you probably already have a good idea as to whether Candida is interfering with your health.

Another very effective and free home test is called the "spit test." I realize this sounds gross, but it's very helpful.

Here's how you do it:

1. Before going to bed put a clear glass of water on your nightstand or dresser. Make sure the container is glass and not plastic or metal because you'll need to see through it.

2. First thing in the morning, briefly rinse your mouth, swallow, then gather some saliva in your mouth from under your tongue and spit into the glass of water (be sure to spit out saliva, not mucus.)

3. Leave the glass undisturbed for 30 - 60 minutes and check back to see if anything has changed. If you see any of the following it indicates that yeast is present:

- Your saliva stayed at the top and there are thin strands that look like strings extending downward.

- Your saliva floats to the bottom and looks cloudy.

- Your saliva is suspended in the middle of the glass, and looks like little specs are floating.

Any of these shows you have an overgrowth of yeast. It's tricky to combat, but once you have it under control you'll feel so much better. Until then it will take time, patience, and perseverance.

Candida Diet Cleanse

———

THIS IS ONE OF THE most effective ways of removing the Candida fungus from your system once and for all. It's a three-stage method designed to do two things:

1. Starve the Fungus

Many of the foods we love eating are the very ones this fungus loves too: sugar, refined carbs, and mold (such as in many cheeses.) The best way to kill this yeast is to starve it—which means not eating these foods.

2. Eliminate Allergens and Sensitivities

Candida easily takes over when the immune system is weak. The problem is, not many people know what they're allergic or sensitive to. That's why following a Candida diet and doing the cleanse is so important. It will help you discover where your weaknesses are.

Is the diet cleanse difficult and expensive?

The most difficult part of the Candida cleanse is starting it since you'll change your way of eating and need to avoid certain foods. Once you get the hang of it though you'll find that it's easy. It can cost as much or as little as you dictate. If you're used to buying a lot of prepared and prepackaged foods, a Candida health plan will probably be cheaper than what you currently spend on meals.

Phase One

Phase one is the most important part if you want to regain your health. This is the stage where you attack Candida by taking away the foods it feeds on and focus on killing the fungus. These are the foods you'll need to stop eating while on the Candida cleanse:

- Sugar (including most fruits, fruit juice, and sweeteners)

- Carbohydrates (simple, complex, all of them)

- Starches (breads, pastas, white rice, etc.)

- Yeast (in breads, beer, etc.)

- Mold (such as in cheeses)

- Gluten

- Wheat

- Dairy (except plain yogurt with live cultures)

- Fermented foods (such as soy sauce and alcohol)

Some Candida diets say that whole grains like amaranth, quinoa, brown rice, buckwheat and millet; low sugar fruits like grapefruit, Granny Smith apples, and berries; and unsweetened yogurt containing live cultures are fine at this stage. On the other hand, some Candida diets say to avoid these.

If you can, avoid them all while on phase one of the cleanse. However, if you can't live without one or more of these foods feel free to enjoy them in small amounts. In my own cleanse I included lemons, Granny Smith apples, and plain yogurt while doing my cleanse and I did well. Just be certain to pay attention to your body. It will tell if something is good or bad, or if it's working or not.

Phase Two

At this point you'll slowly add foods back to your diet. Only add one food at a time so you don't overload your digestive system, and to know if you have a reaction to that food. After each addition it's important to note whether you feel any reaction, even if it's your heart rate going up, a headache, bloating, or gas.

Keeping a food diary is a good idea during all stages. Just write down exactly what you ate and drank each time something passes your lips, and then make notes of how you feel afterward. Check in with your body after consuming anything after 5 minutes, 15 minutes, *and* 30 minutes. Over time you'll see what foods and beverages make you feel energetic and which ones make you feel lethargic or sick.

I recently discovered that rye bread makes me itchy from head to toes. I don't have bread often, but do love rye bread toast occasionally. At first, I couldn't figure out why I had been feeling so itchy, so started back with my food diary.

Sure enough, about half an hour after eating the rye bread the itching would start. If I hadn't kept the diary that toast would have been long-forgotten after half an hour and I'd still be wondering why I felt the way I did.

Phase Three

At this stage you've reintroduced more foods and can resume some sort of normal diet. You've hopefully discovered which foods you're allergic or sensitive to and avoid them altogether or have them only rarely.

Through my own Candida experience and keeping the food diary, I've found that I can't have artificial sweeteners at all. Not because they contribute to Candida, but because they give me anxiety attacks. I also can't have potatoes, caffeine, raw onions, egg yolks, tomato sauce, or rye bread because they bother my stomach or skin in some way.

I *can* have them occasionally, but not on an everyday basis. If I had never done the Candida cleanse I'd still be miserable, struggling with my health, and never knowing what foods affected me and in which ways.

How long should each phase last?

This depends on how sick you currently are. I stayed on phase one for a couple of months, and phase two even longer. Of course, I was very ill and overrun with Candida, so it took a long while to heal.

You might not have to stay on each phase for as long as I did, though two weeks to a month on phase one is a good rule of thumb since this is the time when you're really attacking the Candida and clearing out your system. Phase two can be another two weeks to a month. Phase three should have you eating normally. Again, just listen to your body.

Starting the Diet Cleanse

———

AS YOU START YOUR CANDIDA Cleanse, here are some things to follow:

- Make an appointment to see your health care professional before starting any diet or health plan.

- Stock up on foods you like and are listed on the Candida diet list. (A detailed list is included in the next few pages.)

- Throw out anything that isn't on the list and may be high in starch and sugar. Your family will benefit from this diet as well, so don't feel bad, as if you're depriving them of "good" foods. If you can't get rid of foods they enjoy, keep them separate from your things so you can easily reach

for healthy foods that will help you heal rather than things that will feed the yeast.

- Don't let yourself get hungry or you'll be tempted to cheat and eat something off-limits. By eating three meals a day and healthy snacks you'll avoid the temptation to consume Candida-feeding foods and be able to stick to your health plan much easier.

- Use your favorite recipes, swapping off-limit food items with ones on the Candida food list. Or, look online and find recipes you and your family will enjoy. You'd be surprised at how delicious Candida diet recipes are. I've included some books and websites in the resources section.

- This isn't a low-calorie diet so there are no limits as to how much you can eat, just be sure you stick to the foods on the Candida diet cleanse list. Simply eat when you're hungry and stop when you're satisfied. If you need to lose weight, you'll most likely shed pounds without even trying once you start eating healthier and killing off the Candida.

Candida Diet Time-frame

If your Candida symptoms are mild, follow the Candida diet and eat from the list of foods for two weeks. If you have moderate to severe symptoms, staying on the Candida diet for two months or longer will be your best bet.

People who have been fighting with yeast infections for years may choose to eat only Candida diet foods indefinitely, adding a few changes over time. This is what I do for the most part. I typically follow a Candida diet plan 5 - 6 days a week then eat whatever I want—in moderation—1 or 2 days a week.

The foods on the list are healthy and well tolerated by most people.

After being on the Candida cleanse diet for a few weeks you should feel more energetic, have a more positive mood, and improved mental focus as well.

Diet Cleanse Foods

WHETHER YOU'RE AN OMNIVORE, pescatarian, vegetarian, or vegan, you can still eat well on the Candida diet. When reading the list of foods below, always keep in mind your personal beliefs, your reaction to various foods, likes and dislikes. I've had friends ranging from vegans, Kosher, Halal, and hardcore carnivores do well on the diet.

The only people who have found the food list tough to stick with are those who are used to lots of overly processed and junk foods, and loads of sugar. However, I feel these people need this diet the most!

Protein List:

Eat protein with each meal since it will help keep you feel full longer and assist the body in healing, while increasing energy levels. While on a Candida plan it's normal to feel low energy in the beginning, so be sure to add plenty of healthy proteins to your diet.

Omnivore proteins:

- Lean meats

- Poultry

- All items on the pescatarian, vegetarian, and vegan lists.

Pescatarian proteins:

- Fish

- Seafood

- All items on the vegetarian and vegan lists

Vegetarian proteins:

- Eggs

- Plain yogurt with live active cultures

- All items on the Vegan list.

Vegans proteins:

- Nuts

- Seeds

- Nut butters

- Beans

- Legumes

- Soy

<u>*Vegetable List:*</u>

All vegetables eaten while on this diet should be low on the glycemic scale. Because these vegetables are low in starch, they won't feed the Candida.

- Artichokes and artichoke hearts

- Asparagus

- Bamboo shoots

- Bean sprouts

- Broccoli

- Brussels sprouts

- Cabbage (green, bok choy, Chinese)

- Carrots (raw, not cooked)

- Cauliflower

- Celery

- Cucumber

- Daikon

- Eggplant

- Leeks

- Greens (collard, kale, mustard, turnip)

- Mushrooms

- Okra

- Onions

- Pea pods

- Peppers

- Radishes

- Salad greens (chicory, endive, escarole, iceberg lettuce, romaine, spinach, arugula, radicchio)

- Squash (yellow/summer/crookneck

- Sugar snap peas

- Swiss chard

- Tomato

- Water chestnuts

- Watercress

- Zucchini

Avoid starchy vegetables like corn, potatoes, cooked carrots, winter squashes, sweet potatoes, and yams since they turn into sugar in the system and feed the yeast. Vegetables low on the glycemic index starve Candida to death then absorb the toxins from the dead yeast, eliminating them from the body.

Fruit List:

Since nearly all fruits are high in natural sugar, they're either completely eliminated or greatly reduced while on the Candida diet, though most people do well on the following fruits.

- Granny Smith apples (no other types of apples)

- Grapefruit

- Lemons

- Limes

- Cranberries

- Strawberries

- Raspberries

- All other berries

- Coconut (unsweetened)

Avoid all fruit juices since they're high in natural sugar and feed yeast.

Dairy List:

- Butter

- Ghee

- Plain Kefir

- Plain Yogurt

Nuts and Seeds List: (low mold)

A lot of nuts—like peanuts, pistachios, and cashews—can have mold. This just aggravates your symptoms and provides Candida with more of what it wants. The following nuts and seeds are considered safe to eat:

Almonds

Coconut (unsweetened)

Flax seed

Hazelnuts

Walnuts

Pecans

Sunflower seeds

Legumes List:

This is a gray area when it comes to a Candida cleanse. Some experts say legumes are fine while others talk as if they're the kiss of death. They're so full of fiber and protein that it's a shame to give them up, especially if your vegan. I follow a mostly vegetarian diet and eat vegan meals frequently. In my personal experience, I did fine with legumes in my diet. However, you might want to limit them to just 2-3 times per week or omit them completely in the beginning. As always, see how your body reacts.

- Lentils

- Peas

- Beans

Grains List:

Stick to low glycemic grains while on the Candida diet since they help to keep blood sugar levels even, have more fiber, and starve yeast. In the beginning you may want to eliminate all grains.

- Amaranth

- Buckwheat

- Millet

- Oat bran

- Quinoa

- Spelt

- Teff

Not everyone can eat grains while on the Candida diet as it can make symptoms worse. The above grains have the least side effects, but see how you do when eating them. While following phase one I avoided all grains, and even now tend to stick with only quinoa and brown rice for the most part. See how well you do on the any of these grains if you decide to incorporate them into your Candida health plan. However, it's best to avoid all grains for the first two weeks at least.

Herbs, Spices, Condiments List:

- Apple cider vinegar

- Basil

- Black pepper

- Bragg's Liquid Aminos (great substitute for fermented soy sauce)

- Cinnamon

- Cloves

- Coconut aminos (great substitute for fermented soy sauce)

- Dill

- Garlic

- Ginger

- Oregano

- Paprika

- Rosemary

- Salt

- Thyme

- Turmeric

Beverage List:

It's important to stay hydrated and flush the dead yeast from your system. Doing so will help to ease many of the Candida die-off symptoms such as headaches and constipation.

- Water: The best beverage of all, it helps to rehydrate your body, reduces headaches, and flushes out toxins. A great morning "body flush" is to drink a glass of warm water with a tablespoon of lemon juice and a packet of no calorie sweetener mixed in.

- Herbal teas: Drink these plain or with no calorie sweetener, hot or iced. Peppermint is one of the best to help kill off Candida.

- Unsweetened cranberry juice: This isn't the same as the typical cranberry juices you find in the store. Those have apple, and/or high fructose corn syrup added. Unsweetened cranberry juice can be found at most health food stores (such as Whole Foods and Trader Joe's) and it's **_very_** sour! A little goes a long way. You can sweeten it by adding one teaspoon (yes, one teaspoon!) of unsweetened cranberry juice to 8oz of water and adding no calorie sweetener to taste.

- Lemonade: Made with 8oz water, one tablespoon of lemon juice and one or two

packets of no-calorie sweetener.

- Chicory coffee: A lot of experts says to avoid coffee while on a Candida cleanse. Chicory "coffee" (such as Postum) is considered okay on the diet though. I'll admit, I couldn't give up my "normal" coffee, but greatly reduced it to just one cup in the morning. I take mine black, but feel free to add a no-calorie sweetener and just a touch of milk or cream if you can tolerate it.

Sweeteners List:

- Splenda

- Equal

- Sweet n' Low

- Erythritol

- Stevia

- Xylitol

Cut out *all* sugar, honey, molasses, agave, you name it. Only no-calorie sweeteners are allowed on this diet. If they don't bother you then go ahead and use them, but I've found that they give me headaches and anxiety attacks. For me, Stevia is fine though, and I haven't had a problem with it. Use your judgment and use everything in moderation.

Fats List:

Fats should be used in moderation since they're high in calories.

- Olive oil

- Canola oil

- Grape seed oil

- Avocado oil

- Flaxseed oil

- Coconut oil

- Butter

- Avocado

- Ghee

- Butter

You can make a somewhat healthier alternative to plain butter by mixing two sticks of room temperature butter with one cup of your chosen oil. Mix well and store in the refrigerator in a bowl with a tight-fitting lid. Use anywhere you would normally use butter.

Booster List:

The following foods and supplements can help boost the effects of your Candida cleanse health plan.

- Garlic

- Oregano

- Lemon juice

- Vitamin C

- Oregano oil capsules

- Grapefruit seed extract tablets or capsules

- Psyllium husk fiber (such as Metamucil)

- Acidophilus

These foods and supplements are excellent at killing the Candida fungus and help to eliminate them from the body. For supplements, take as directed on the bottle.

Eating only from the lists of anti-Candida foods will help to kill off the yeast and eventually restore your health and energy.

Candida Diet Tips

———

AS I MENTIONED IN THE Candida diet cleanse above, you'll need to eliminate all sugars, high-carbohydrate foods and starchy vegetables for a limited time since they feed the yeast. Adding probiotic foods to your diet can be very helpful. When I did the cleanse would eat plain Greek yogurt daily, and still do. You can also eat organic sauerkraut or kimchi before any meal to get your digestive juices going and help regulate your stomach acid.

You'll probably feel a little (or a lot) low energy for the first few days if you're used to having a lot of sugar and/or carbohydrates. *This is a perfectly normal sign of detoxification.* To combat these feelings, you can eat more good fats (olives, olive oil, avocado, nuts), low carbohydrates vegetables—especially leafy greens—and lean protein.

Prepare homemade salad dressings using olive oil, garlic, lemon juice, and your favorite herbs.

Keep a big bowl of fresh salad in your fridge so you'll have access to healthy food all the time and won't be as tempted to cheat and have something that will set you back on your health plan.

I got so sick of lettuce that I started making chopped salads with chunks of my favorite veggies. Sometimes I added a chopped apple or two that I tossed with lemon juice to prevent browning. Whenever I was hungry I could fill a bowl with the chopped salad and top with my favorite dressing. I'd often add an avocado, or olives, and would sprinkle some nuts on top. It was a complete meal in a bowl!

Another good tip is to cook up a batch of boneless, skinless chicken breasts and/or hard boiled eggs to keep on hand as well. You can chop them up and add them to salads or snack on them when you feel hungry.

The key to making your Candida diet cleanse a success is to make eating as simple as possible. It's so easy to abandon a health plan if you have to spend a lot of time cooking or preparing foods.

Natural Remedies

I LISTED MOST OF THESE on the Candida diet in the boosters list, but I want to go over them in a bit more detail here, so you can see why they're so powerful.

Grapefruit Seed Extract:

Also known as GSE this supplement is one of the strongest *natural* anti-fungals/antibiotics known to man. I always have a bottle of the tablets in my house and use it for everything from Candida and UTIs, to colds.

It can be used in both tablet and liquid form, though I highly recommend the tablets since the liquid is incredibly bitter. Oregano oil works just as well, but it gave me terrible indigestion, which is why I stick with GSE.

Garlic:

This is one of the single best supplements anyone can take. Not only is it effective against Candida and other fungal infections, but it's often recommended to help boost the immune system and for heart health. Use fresh garlic in cooking. As a supplement, take at least 500mg in divided doses up to 3 times per day, or follow package directions.

Probiotics:

These beneficial bacteria produce a natural compound which can oxidize infectious organisms such as Candida Albicans and help to rebalance your intestinal tract. Yogurt, kefir, and organic sauerkraut are examples of probiotic foods. In supplement form look for acidophilus or a combination supplement with several strains for probiotics and take as directed.

Oil of Oregano:

This is an incredibly potent anti-fungal, and is also a great anti-viral and anti-inflammatory as well. If you suspect that you have Candida be sure to add oregano oil to your arsenal list. Available in capsule and liquid form, I prefer capsules since the oil is *very* overpowering. This supplement rapidly destroys Candida while also reducing the damage caused by it. It gave me heartburn though, so I stick with grapefruit seed extract.

Apple Cider Vinegar:

Also called ACV, be sure to buy the organic kind with the "mother", and hasn't been pasteurized with all the good bacteria killed off. I use Bragg's brand.

Organic ACV is especially useful as an external or vaginal wash. One way to use it is to take a bath and add one cup of apple cider vinegar to the water.

It can also be taken internally daily, adding it to salads or consumed in drinks. Every morning I fill a mug with warm water and add a teaspoon or two of ACV and a packet of stevia. Not everyone likes the tastes of vinegar, so feel free to skip the vinegar drink and use it in your salads instead.

Psyllium Fiber:

Unless your doctor recommends otherwise, I fully believe everyone should take a fiber supplement daily. Most people don't get nearly enough fiber in their diets, which leads to chronic constipation and a buildup of gunk in the intestinal tract. I struggled with many intestinal issues, but once I added psyllium fiber they virtually disappeared within just a few days.

Psyllium swells to about five times its original size and makes you feel fuller faster too, which is great if you want to lose weight. This fiber is like a broom and will sweep out your system, carrying Candida—and cholesterol—with it. There are so many benefits that come with taking this supplement that it's foolish not to.

I prefer sugar-free orange flavored Metamucil or the Wal-Mart Equate brand, though some prefer the plain fiber. Other fiber supplements are not psyllium (such as Benefiber) and don't offer the same benefits.

More than diet alone, you'll want to add some or all these natural supplements to your health plan to fully eliminate Candida.

Common Die-Off Symptoms

———

WHILE FOLLOWING YOUR Candida diet cleanse you'll very likely face die-off symptoms. As the yeast is killed it floods the body with toxins and can cause many of the symptoms listed below. Although the list is long, if you experience any of these side-effects it's a positive sign that your body is clearing out the fungal infection. Within a week or two these uncomfortable symptoms will lessen, and your health will dramatically improve.

- Dizziness

- Headache

- Fuzzy thinking

- Depression

- Anxiety

- Angry outbursts

- Gas & bloating

- Diarrhea

- Constipation

- Joint pain

- Muscle pain

- Body aches

- Sore throat

- Fatigue

- Exhaustion

- Need for more sleep

- Sweating

- Chills

- Nausea

- Skin breakouts

Here are some ways to help lessen the Candida die-off symptoms:

Flush It Out

Help your body flush out the Candida Albicans by drinking at least half a gallon to one gallon of water or unsweetened herbal tea each day. It's recommended to not drink any more than one gallon of water unless you're very dehydrated (due to summer heat and/or intense physical exercise) as this can cause an imbalance in the body's electrolytes.

Soak It Out

Add one cup of Epsom salts or baking soda to a bathtub of water as hot as is comfortable. Soak in the tub for up to half an hour to help draw out toxins through the pores of your skin. Don't soak in a hot tub though if you're pregnant.

Sweat it out

Exercising produces sweat, which in turn this helps to release toxins through the body's largest organ: the skin. By exercising 3-6 times a week for 15 or 30 minutes each time, you can assist your body's detoxification efforts, lift your mood, increase energy and health, and strengthen your

muscles.

Supplements Can Help

Vitamins that boost the immune system are helpful in reducing yeast die-off symptoms. Some good choices are vitamins A, C, E, and selenium. Fiber supplements such as psyllium husk or oat fiber will bind to toxins, pulling them from the body through elimination. Take these as directed

on the package labels.

Die-Off Time-frame

The more intense your Candida cleanse program, and the worse your Candida overgrowth is, the more severe your die-off symptoms will be. Prescription drugs such as Nystatin tend to cause the worse die-off symptoms, with natural anti-fungals such as grapefruit seed extract and oregano oil capsules causing slightly less severe symptoms.

Depending on how long you've had Candida will usually determine how long symptoms will last. The average time is approximately two weeks, though everyone heals at their own rate. Mine seemed to last forever, but ultimately, I felt better than ever. Remember, symptoms are only temporary, showing that your cleansing program is working.

Preventing Future Yeast Infections

———

CANDIDA CAN CAUSE MANY uncomfortable symptoms that can be life altering. Once treated, you'll obviously want to avoid any recurring infections. Here are 10 effective tips to prevent future yeast infections:

1. Get Enough Sleep:

Your immune system really suffers from lack of sleep and unhealthy stress, giving Candida the upper hand. Be sure to get at least 8 hours of sleep each night to help keep your immune system strong and prevent a fungus overgrowth.

2. Proper Diet:

As we've discussed, too many starches and carbs and too much sugar can stimulate an overgrowth of bodily yeast. Eat nutritious and healthy foods from the Candida cleanse diet list. Including a daily serving of yogurt with live active cultures can help keep this infection away. You can even follow the Candida diet for the rest of your life, choosing to have a few "cheat" meals here and there.

3. Wear Cotton Underwear:

Remember, Candida thrives in an environment of heat and humidity. It really loves the moist and tight environment of satin, silk, PVC, nylon, lace, leather, latex, lycra, and polyester panties! Cotton underwear allows air circulation and helps prevent yeast overgrowth.

4. Use Water-Based Lubricants:

During intercourse, or even hand manipulation, use water-based products since they don't disturb the natural chemistry of your genitalia.

5. Avoid Perfumed Feminine Products:

Stay away from scented tampons, pads, toilet papers, feminine washes, and creams. These can irritate sensitive areas, upsetting the natural vaginal flora and lead to yeast infections.

6. Limit Antibiotic Use:

Although antibiotics are effective in treating infections, they kill both the bad and good bacteria. This good bacterium keeps yeast growth in-check and without it Candida proliferates. Only use antibiotics when necessary and as prescribed by your doctor.

7. Avoid Douching:

The chemicals used when douching disrupt the pH balance of the vagina, increasing the chances of getting a yeast infection. The vagina is meant to be self-cleaning, but if you must douche, use a gentle vinegar and water solution.

8. Stay Dry:

During the summer, if you sweat a lot, be sure to change your underwear frequently. Also, after showering, exercising, or swimming, make sure to dry off properly before putting your underwear and clothes on. Candida loves warm, damp areas.

9. Before Sex:

Before having sex be certain that you and your partner wash your genitals well. This may cut into any spontaneity and not seem romantic, but it can help you avoid recurring yeast infections. Bacteria on the genitals can be introduced into the vagina leading to an overgrowth of Candida.

10. Change Birth Control:

If you keep getting yeast infections and are on birth control pills, it might be a good idea to switch to a non-hormonal form of birth control. My daughter has this problem and she and her husband now rely on condoms. There are some condoms on the market that are very thin, barely noticeable, and latex-free.

FAQs

I'VE TRIED TO COVER everything I've done and experienced while on my personal Candida healing program, though I've shared some questions friends and clients have asked me over the years.

Is a Candida cleanse the same as a colon cleanse?

When doing your Candida cleanse, it's very helpful to take in more fiber to help flush the toxins from your system, though this is a very small part of the process. A true Candida cleanse is really about using diet and supplements to get rid of the yeast overgrowth. Typically, a colon cleanse focuses only on taking in more fiber or supplements that empty the bowels, though doesn't kill off Candida.

Do I need to watch food portions on this diet?

All you should focus on is the food lists rather than portion sizes. This isn't a weight loss diet where you stick to a certain number of calories each day. You need to keep up your strength and stick to the health plan and eradicate the fungus once and for all. Eat when you're hungry and stop when you're satisfied, it's as simple as that.

Why are some foods restricted?

There are two reasons why certain types of foods are restricted during a Candida cleanse: To starve the fungus of its food source and to remove foods that irritate your immune system. As we talked about earlier in the book, starches and sugars feed yeast, as do moldy foods, some dairy products and gluten. If you starve anything it will die, and that's what you want!

Will I lose weight on this plan?

If you currently need to lose weight, then you'll almost definitely drop pounds while following the Candida diet. After years of eating overly processed and highly fatty foods it's easy to gain and keep the weight. Even so-called diet foods can put on the pounds since they're filled with preservatives and junk ingredients and not real food your body craves. Once you begin eating the foods on the Candida list you'll lose weight without even trying. Your body will find its natural ideal weight and you'll probably feel healthier than you have in a long time.

Do I need to take the supplements too?

I've been asked if it's possible to only follow the Candida diet and omit the supplements. If you've been suffering with yeast infection symptoms for some time, I highly recommend taking at least 2-3 supplements from the list. I found the most relief with a psyllium fiber drink each morning, taking grapefruit seed extract twice a day, and a probiotic.

I took both acidophilus capsules and ate a serving of plain Greek yogurt daily. These seemed to be most gentle on my system yet knocked out the Candida quickly. Dieting alone isn't the best option when trying to heal.

What about side effects?

I mentioned Candida die-off symptoms earlier, also called Herxheimer response. There are very few people who won't experience symptoms to one degree or another since it's a natural part of the fungus dying and being flushed from the body. While the Candida are alive they produce toxic chemicals as a byproduct. When the fungi die, they flood the body with these toxins which can cause an immediate worsening of symptoms.

This is the point where many people want to stop a Candida cleanse. They want to get better not worse! Please stick with the program though since this is a positive sign, showing that the Candida is leaving your body.

Symptoms can last anywhere from a couple of days to two weeks or longer, and this is where fiber drinks (like Metamucil) come in handy. They help to flush these toxins out of your system quickly. Taking extra supplements like vitamin C can also help with side effects and keep your immune system strong.

Other questions?

Although I'm not a medical doctor or Candida expert, I *have* been down this road a few times and will gladly answer any questions you have or offer moral support while you're on this path. I know how confusing and frustrating it can be!

AuthorKellyWallace@gmail.com

Resources

THESE ARE SOME OF THE books and websites I've found to be most helpful. However, I urge you to educate yourself and seek out other books and websites I haven't included. Also, over the years some websites are no longer available, information changes, and books become hard to find.

Websites:

CandidaMD.com (Candida symptoms)

BodyEcology.com (Candida quiz)

NaturalNews.com (Candida natural remedies)

YeastConnection.com (Lots of great information about Candida and curing it.)

LowCarbFriends.com (Forum with lots of anti-Candida recipes)

IHerb.com (This is where I buy my supplements. They're typically cheaper than the stores.)

Books:

The Yeast Connection - William Crook

Complete Candida Yeast Guidebook - Jeanne Marie Martin

Chronic Candidiasis - Michael T. Murray

The Candida Control Cookbook - Gail Burton

The Body Ecology Diet - Donna Gates and Linda Schatz

The Bible Cure for Candida and Yeast Infections - Donald Colbert

Contact Me/Book A Reading

WHETHER YOUR PROBLEMS or concerns are in the areas of love, finances, family, career, health, education, or your path in life, I offer professional psychic counseling, caring guidance, and solutions that work!

I use no tools. Instead, I'll connect directly with your higher self and your spirit guides to help you through any situation and achieve the best possible results. No problem is too big or too small, and your questions will be answered in detail.

I'll let you know absolutely everything that comes through in the reading which typically includes past, present, and future energies, guidance, time frames and predictions. Your guides may also include information on an important past life, aura energy, soul symbols, and more. Each reading is in-depth, filled with positive energy and guidance, and includes one free clarification email.

All readings are done via email. By offering my readings through email you'll be able to save your reading and go back to it again and again for guidance.

I look forward to reading for you!

Check out my readings, books, blog posts, and more on my website:

DrKellyPsychic.com

Or email me directly at: DrKellyPsychicCounselor@gmail.com

Don't miss out!

Visit the website below and you can sign up to receive emails whenever Kelly Wallace publishes a new book. There's no charge and no obligation.

https://books2read.com/r/B-A-CIDB-PIBE

BOOKS 2 READ

Connecting independent readers to independent writers.

Did you love *How To Cure Candida - Yeast Infection Causes, Symptoms, Diet & Natural Remedies*? Then you should read *The Power Of Pets*[1] by Kelly Wallace!

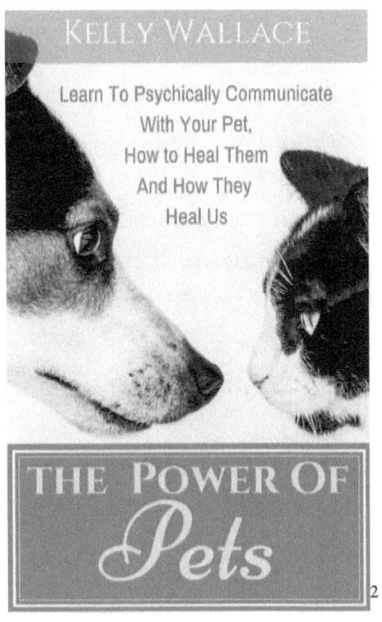

[2]

Many people seek the help of "animal whisperers". These professionals seem to have a natural knack for intuitively knowing what animals want and need. They can find out if a pet is ill, why they have certain behavioral problems, what the pet thinks of their owners, and how to make your furry loved one happier and healthier. But, more and more people are realizing that they can psychically or intuitively communicate with their pets themselves.

1. https://books2read.com/u/bP56Zl

2. https://books2read.com/u/bP56Zl

If you've had pets, I'm sure you can see how different their personalities were. I bet you'll smile at your memories of them too. Pets can bring us so much joy. They can also help us heal, just as we can help them. You can even learn to communicate with them—whether your furry family member is in this world or the after world.

Pets have so much to say to us, but first you need to tune into them to understand the messages they're sending. Learning to read their body language is simple, and as you get more accustomed to this you can even communicate telepathically! That might sound incredible, but you'll be surprised at how easy it is. Since various animals have different levels of consciousness they'll communicate on their own unique level. In time you'll learn how your pet communicates what it wants you to know. I'll show you how!

Read more at psychicreadingsbydrkelly.webs.com.

Also by Kelly Wallace

Upgrade Your Life - Small Changes Easy Actions Big Success

10 Minutes A Day To A Powerful New Life!

Healing The Child Within

Is He The One? Finding And Keeping Your Soulmate

True Wealth - Reprogram Your Subconscious For Financial Success

Best Friends Better Lovers

Looking For Mr. Right

No-Sweat Homeschooling

Psychic Vampires - Protect and Heal Yourself From Energy Predators

Spirit Guides And Healing Energy

Cowboys Make Better Lovers

Hellraiser

Intuitive Tarot - Learn The Tarot Instantly

One Wicked Night

Chakra Energy

Contacting Your Spirit Guides - Meeting and Working With Your Invisible Helpers

Energy Work - Heal, Cleanse, And Strengthen Your Aura

Clear Your Karma - The Healing Power Of Your Past Lives

Intuitive Living - Developing Your Psychic Gifts

Animal Magnetism - Bad Boys Gone Good

Confessions - Everyone Has A Secret At Ryder Ranch

Passion And Parsecs

Two In The Bush

Become Your Higher Self

The Art Of Happiness

Creating A Charmed Life

Wrong Brother Right Lover

The Power Of Pets

Working With Your Angels
Transforming Your Money Mindset
Spiritual Alchemy
Master The Art Of: Picking Up Women, Sex & Seduction, Dating Women (3 books in 1)
Finding Your Life Purpose - Uncover Your Soul's True Goals
DreamWork: Using The Wisdom Of Your Sleeping Mind To Change Your Waking Life
The Mended Soul - Healing Your Mind, Body, & Spirit From Anxiety & Depression
The Overwhelmed Empath - A Guide For Sensitive Souls
Breaking The Worry Habit - Stop Your Anxious Thoughts And Start Living!
Shadow Work: Understanding and Making Peace With Your Darker Side
Never Good Enough - Escaping The Prison Of Perfectionism
Signs From The Universe
Way Of The Lightworker
One Wicked Night

Watch for more at psychicreadingsbydrkelly.webs.com.